FOOD REMEDY FOR HIGH BLOOD PRESSURE

18 First Class Foods for High Blood Pressure

Harry James

Table of Contents

CHAPTER I 3

   Description 3

   What Is Blood Pressure?...........3

   What Are Ordinary Blood Pressure Numbers?....................5

   What Is Excessive Blood Pressure (High Blood Pressure)? 5

   What causes high blood pressure? 8

CHAPTER II....................................9

   18 First-Class Foods for High Blood Pressure 9

   18 Ingredients That Help Lower Blood Pressure 11

THE END 32

CHAPTER I

Description

What Is Blood Pressure?

Blood pressure is the stress of blood pushing in opposition to the partitions of your arteries. Arteries deliver blood from your coronary heart to different parts of your body.

Your blood pressure generally rises and falls all through the day.

What Do Blood Pressure Numbers Imply?

Blood pressure is measured the usage of numbers:

The first wide variety, called systolic blood pressure, measures the pressure in your arteries whilst your heart beats.

The 2d number, known as diastolic blood pressure, measures the pressure in your arteries when your heart rests among beats.

If the size reads a 120 and 80 diastolic, you would say, "one hundred twenty over 80," or write, "one hundred twenty/80 mmHg."

What Are Ordinary Blood Pressure Numbers?

A normal blood pressure level is much less than 120/80 mmHg.1

No count your age, you can take steps every day to hold your blood pressure in a healthy range.

What Is Excessive Blood Pressure (High Blood Pressure)?

High blood pressure, additionally called hypertension, is blood pressure this is better than every day. Your blood pressure adjustments at some point of the day based in your activities.

Having blood pressure measures constantly above ordinary may additionally bring about an analysis of high blood strain (or high blood pressure).

The better your blood pressure tiers, the more risk you have for different health issues, together with coronary heart disorder, coronary heart assault, and stroke.

Your health care group can diagnose excessive blood pressure and make remedy selections through reviewing your systolic and diastolic blood pressure degrees and comparing them to tiers located in positive guidelines.

The guidelines used to diagnose high blood pressure may additionally differ from health care expert to health care expert:

• Some fitness care professionals diagnose sufferers with excessive blood stress if their blood strain is continuously 140/90 mm Hg or better.2 this limit is based on a guideline launched in 2003, as visible in the table underneath.

• Other fitness care experts diagnose sufferers with high blood stress if their blood pressure is continuously 130/80 mm Hg or better.

What causes high blood pressure?

High blood pressure usually develops over time. It can happen because of unhealthy lifestyle choices, such as not getting enough regular physical activity. Certain health conditions, such as diabetes and having obesity, can also increase the risk for developing high blood pressure. High blood pressure can also happen during pregnancy.

CHAPTER II

18 First-Class Foods for High Blood Pressure

Research has proven that certain foods — which includes fruits, veggies, nuts, and oily fish — can decrease blood strain. Combining those meals in the food regimen might also result in lengthy-time period health advantages.

Medications, dietary adjustments, and different way of life changes can lessen excessive blood strain, or high blood pressure, at the same time as decreasing the likelihood of developing associated conditions. High blood strain increases someone's risk of coronary heart ailment, stroke, and kidney disorder.

Types of meals which can assist consist of:

- Culmination, which includes kiwi and oranges

- Vegetables, for instance, inexperienced leafy veggies and beets

- Nuts, as an example, pistachios and walnuts

- Oily fish, along with mackerel

- Spices, along with cinnamon

This article discusses ingredients which can help reduce high blood strain and provide medical proof.

18 Ingredients That Help Lower Blood Pressure

1. Berries

Blueberries and strawberries incorporate antioxidant compounds called anthocyanins, a form of flavonoid.

To Experience Berries:

•   consume them as a snack or candy treat after meals

•   upload them to smoothies

•   sprinkle them on oatmeal for breakfast

• A serving of blueberries is around 1 cup of sparkling or frozen blueberries or half of a cup of dried blueberries. A serving of strawberries is around 7 strawberries.

• Which different meals are rich in antioxidants?

2. Bananas

• Bananas contain potassium that may help manipulate high blood pressure. One medium-sized banana includes round 422 milligrams (mg) Trusted Source of potassium.

- A serving might be 1 huge banana, 1 cup of sliced banana, or -thirds of a cup of mashed banana.

An adult males purpose to devour 3-4 hundred mg of potassium every day and adult females — 2,600 mg.

Other potassium-wealthy meals include:

- Apricots

- Lentils

- Prunes

- Acorn squash

- Potatoes

People with kidney disease should consult a physician earlier than growing their potassium consumption, as too much can be harmful.

3. Beets

Drinking beet juice may additionally reduce blood stress within the brief and long time because it includes dietary nitrate.

According to a 2022 systematic studies indicates that nitrate from beetroot juice lowers systolic blood stress in people with arterial high blood pressure however does no longer have an effect on diastolic blood stress.

Tips To Be Used Include:

• consuming 1 glass of beet juice in line with day

• including beets to salads

• getting ready beets as a facet dish

A serving of beet is around 1 cup of raw, cooked, or juiced beets.

4. Dark Chocolate

Cacao, an aspect in dark chocolate, contains flavonoids, an antioxidant. Flavonoids might also help reduce blood pressure, in step with the AHA.

However, it notes that someone might not be capable of devour enough flavonoids in dark chocolate to experience vast benefits.

The AHA says that a small quantity of chocolate now and again may be a part of a balanced weight loss plan. It advises, but, that human beings eat it due to the fact they experience it, not for fitness reasons.

5. Kiwis

A day by day serving of kiwi can lessen systolic blood stress, among other benefits.

People who ate 2 kiwis in step with day earlier than breakfast for 7 weeks had a discount of 2.7 millimeters of mercury (mmHg) in systolic blood pressure compared to a manage organization.

Kiwis also are rich in diet C. vitamin C supplementation drastically decreased blood pressure in people with primary hypertension.

Kiwis are easy to feature to lunches or smoothies. One cup of kiwi, or 2–3 kiwifruits, makes up 1 serving.

6. Watermelon

Watermelon incorporates an amino acid called citrulline.

The body converts citrulline to arginine, and this allows the frame produce nitric oxide, a gasoline that relaxes blood vessels and encourages flexibility in arteries. These results useful resource blood drift that can decrease excessive blood stress.

A small 2023 controlled crossover trial checked out the effects of watermelon juice on blood strain in young, healthy adults. They found that watermelon juice lowered systolic blood strain over two hours.

27 people fed on either watermelon juice or another drink earlier than exercise. The females who drank watermelon juice did now not enjoy a upward thrust in blood pressure after workout, even though the men did.

People can consume watermelon:

- As juice

- In salads, along with fruit salads

- In smoothies

- In a chilled watermelon soup

One serving of watermelon is 1 cup of chopped fruit or 1 slice of round 2 inches.

7. Oats

Oats include a sort of fiber called beta-glucan, which can also benefit coronary heart health, inclusive of blood stress.

These effects recommend that components found in oats can help prevent excessive blood pressure and protect coronary heart fitness in different methods. However, in addition studies on human subjects is necessary.

Ways of eating oats consist of:

• having a bowl of oatmeal for breakfast

- The use of rolled oats in preference to breadcrumbs to present texture to burger patties

- sprinkling them on yogurt cakes

8. Leafy Green Vegetables

Leafy green greens are wealthy in nitrates, which assist manage blood pressure.

Research from 2021Trusted Source indicates that ingesting at the least 1 cup of green leafy veggies day by day can decrease blood strain and reduce the chance of cardiovascular disease.

Examples of leafy veggies consist of:

- Cabbage

- Collard vegetables

- Kale

- Mustard greens

- Spinach

- Swiss chard

To consume a everyday dose of green veggies, someone can:

- stir spinach into curries and stews

- Sauté Swiss chard with garlic as a facet dish

- bake a batch of kale chips

A serving of fresh leafy greens is two cups of clean leaves or 1 cup of cooked leafy veggies.

9. Garlic

Garlic has antibiotic and antifungal properties, lots of which can be due to its principal energetic factor, allicin.

Garlic, can reduce:

- Blood stress

- Arterial stiffness

- Cholesterol

Garlic can enhance the taste of many savory food, inclusive of stir-fries, soups, and omelets. It also can be an alternative to salt as a flavoring.

10. Fermented Meals

Fermented meals are rich in probiotics, which might be beneficial microorganism that could help manage blood stress.

Sodium is a risk thing for excessive blood strain, and experts Fermented ingredients to feature to the food regimen encompass:

- Kimchi

- Kombucha

- Apple cider vinegar

- Miso

- Tempeh

Probiotic supplements are any other choice.

11. Lentils and Different Pulses

Lentils offer protein and fiber, and benefit the blood vessels of people with high blood pressure.

Legume consumption of fifty five–70 grams (g) each day with a decrease threat of hypertension. Legumes included lentils, peas, beans, and more.

People can use lentils in lots of approaches, consisting of:

- As an opportunity to minced beef

- including bulk to salads

- As a base for stews and soups

12. Natural Yogurt

Yogurt is fermented dairy food.

The contributors with excessive blood stress who fed on extra yogurt had lower systolic blood pressure and decrease arterial strain than folks who did no longer.

To enjoy unsweetened yogurt:

- add 1 spoonful to a plate of stew or curry

- Mix with chopped cucumber, mint, and garlic as a side dish

- use it rather than cream on fruit and desserts

- spoon it onto an aggregate of oatmeal, nuts, and dried fruit for breakfast

13. Pomegranates

Pomegranates contain antioxidants and other substances that may help prevent excessive blood strain and atherosclerosis.

A 2018 trial suggests that each day pomegranate juice consumption may reduce systolic and diastolic blood stress in people with diabetes. However, the authors stress the want for further studies.

People can consume pomegranates complete or as juice. When shopping for prepackaged pomegranate juice, test to make sure that there may be no delivered sugar.

14. Cinnamon

Cinnamon may additionally help lessen blood stress by means of a modest quantity. The authors found that eating up to 2 g of cinnamon day by day for eight weeks or more decreased blood pressure in humans with a frame mass index (BMI) of 30 or more.

To include cinnamon into the weight-reduction plan, a person can:

- upload it to oatmeal as an alternative to sugar

- sprinkle it on freshly chopped fruit

- upload it to smoothies

15. Nuts

Several research have located that eating nuts of various kinds can help control high blood pressure.

A 2019 studyTrusted Source shows ordinary walnut consumption reduces systolic blood stress in older adults with mind hypertension.

A 2022 pass-sectional examine also suggests that moderate nut consumption, fifty five–a hundred g day by day, can also help to control high blood pressure in children.

Opt for unsalted nuts and:

- Snack on them undeniable

- upload them to salads

- Mixture them into pestos

- use them in essential dishes, such as nut roast

People must now not eat nuts in the event that they have a nut hypersensitive reaction.

THE END

www.ingramcontent.com/pod-product-compliance
Lightning Source LLC
Chambersburg PA
CBHW060018300526
45794CB00003B/1213